Background

Today, a confluence of events is compelling the health care industry to closely examine its employment and training practices. Health care reform, the aging of the "baby boomer" population and advances in technology have all triggered a need for a paradigm shift relative to workforce planning. Health care occupations dominate the list of jobs predicted to be in most demand in coming years, and there is simply not enough talent in the pipeline.

People with disabilities have an important role to play in meeting the demands of a rapidly changing health care landscape. Not only can this population assist in responding to looming workforce shortages, it offers significant value and insight that can improve care. However, the employment rate of people with disabilities in health care occupations remains unacceptably low due to a range of barriers, both architectural and attitudinal.

Reflecting these realities, DOL's Office of Disability Employment Policy (ODEP), under the leadership of Assistant Secretary Kathy Martinez and in conjunction with Access Living of Metropolitan Chicago, convened the *Health Care: Career Trends, Best Practices & Call-to-Action Summit* on May 17, 2011. Nearly 100 people participated in the invitation-only event, representing a diverse cross-section of stakeholders including health care professionals with disabilities, government agencies, service providers, business leaders, researchers and advocates from across the country (for a list of participants, see Appendix A: Participant List).

In addition to the rich dialogue that transpired, the event itself was a milestone, marking the first time DOL/ODEP gathered thought leaders together to specifically explore the intersection between disability employment and health care — an industry at a historic crossroads and of consequence to all Americans.

Welcome

Brief summary: Five leaders from the health care and disability communities, both in Chicago and nationally, welcomed participants and shared their vision for disability employment in the health care industry in the context of their overall work.

Access Living Chairman of the Board Eric Grossman welcomed everyone, noting that employment is a critical component of Access Living's commitment to fostering an inclusive society that enables people with disabilities to live fully engaged, self-directed lives. He gave a brief history of Access Living, sharing that its universally designed building was opened in 2007 with the support of former Mayor Daley. He also encouraged everyone to take a few minutes after the event to tour the building and meet the organization's staff.

Rush University Medical Center CEO Dr. Larry Goodman thanked everyone for coming and said he felt that Access Living was a most appropriate venue for discussion issues related to disability and employment, given its President and CEO Marca Bristo's history of leadership on the issue, both locally and globally. He then shared information about his organization's involvement, noting a number of actionable examples, including an ADA taskforce; a 2003 symposium focused on technical standards and how they may negatively impact employment and educational opportunities for people with disabilities; and a partnership with National Louis University to provide fellowships to adults with autism. He added that Rush University Medical Center has been recognized for excellence in this area, but that he'll really know they've made a difference when there is no such need for awards, because good workplace practices for people with disabilities are routine.

Commissioner of the City of Chicago Mayor's Office for People with Disabilities Karen Tamley said she was pleased to be back at Access Living, where she worked as Director of Programs prior to being appointed to her current position by former Mayor Daley and now reappointed by current Mayor Emanuel. She said that her office works to meet the diverse needs of people with disabilities who live and work in Chicago, with the goal of making it the most accessible city in the nation. She said this goal incorporates employment, including job exploration and competitive internship programs for city high school students with disabilities that focus on not just jobs, but long-term careers, such as those in the health care arena.

Assistant Secretary of Labor for Disability Employment Policy Kathleen Martinez welcomed participants and noted that this event was second in a series of industry "sector summits" sponsored by ODEP in conjunction with advocacy organizations such as Access Living across the nation; the first focused on entertainment and media. She then introduced Secretary of Labor Hilda Solis, noting her strong support of ODEP's work since she assumed her position in early 2009 and dedication to weaving disability into the fabric of all DOL programs and services, as opposed to treating it as a separate issue.

Secretary of Labor Hilda L. Solis said she was pleased to be in Chicago, both because it is known for being a hub of health care innovation and because it reminds her of her home state of California, where she worked on health care as well as disability issues as a state legislator and then congressperson. She added that she is proud to be part of the disability movement, and that she hoped the day's discussions would result in actionable ideas for advancing her vision of "good jobs for everyone" by making workplaces accessible for those who want to train and work in health care. She also said that the disability community has an ally in President Obama, and recognized Eric Grossman, Dr. Goodman and Kareem Dale for their support, in addition to Assistant Secretary Martinez. She also noted another disability champion, Senator Tom Harkin (D-IA), and encouraged people to reach out to him.

Secretary Solis acknowledged that disability issues aren't always easy, because often they require advocating for more money, and that some policymakers avoid related committees and initiatives as a result. As a result, it's essential for the disability community to amplify its voice and make sure elected officials don't take budget battles out on vulnerable populations, which is what is occurring with the tax imposed by some states with regards to the Affordable Care Act, she said.

Under her leadership, disability is not a separate issue at DOL, Secretary Solis said, noting that she has strong support from not only Assistant Secretary Martinez but also Director of the Office of Federal Contract Compliance Programs (OFCCP) Patricia Shiu, who helps enforce DOL's laws and ensure tax dollars are not used to discriminate. In addition, over the past two years, DOL has also significantly invested in training in high-demand industries, including health care and, just recently, information technology (IT) through the H-1B technical skills training grant competition.

Secretary Solis said that for far too long, people with disabilities have been perceived as those only on the receiving end of health care, despite evidence that that people with disabilities have the skills to work at all levels in the industry. In recent weeks, the Social Security Board of Trustees released its 2011 annual report on the financial health of the Social Security Trust Funds (combined assets of the Old-Age and Survivors Insurance and Disability Insurance Trust Funds), and this discussion drew attention to the fact that investing in getting people jobs is one obvious solution to the projected exhaustion of the Disability Insurance Trust Fund in 2018.

Secretary Solis closed by sharing that as a child, she was misdiagnosed as having a learning disability when in fact she had low vision. As a result, she said, some people began to "write her off," and she would not be where she is today if other people hadn't advocated on her behalf. Thus, she wants to make sure young people, especially those from low-income immigrant families, can get the services they need to learn and prepare for a meaningful career. Reflecting this, she expressed sincere appreciation for the work of summit participants, today and into the future.

Associate Director, White House Office of Public Engagement & Special Assistant to the President for Disability Policy Kareem Dale noted that since assuming his position, he has been communicating frequently with Assistant Secretary Martinez because her work is critical to one of President Obama's top priorities, getting people, including people with disabilities, back to work. People with disabilities must have a seat at the table and an opportunity to shine and reach the American dream, he said. In addition, the Obama Administration is committed to letting citizens participate in and influence the policymaking process, as evidenced by this summit, he said. He added that another mechanism for facilitating this engagement process is the monthly Disability Calls and White House disability web page. He asked those in the room not already involved in the ongoing dialogue to join it, and for those already involved to invite others in. He also said he looked forward to another great summer celebrating the anniversary of the ADA and Olmstead decision.

Assistant Secretary Martinez then summarized the topics to be discussed throughout the rest of the summit, dubbing it the "no excuses" day, because it was a time to focus not on the problem, but its solutions, and for tackling not only barriers that are architectural, but also attitudinal. With people from all parts of the puzzle, there should be no shortage of ideas for improving employment opportunities for people with disabilities in the health care field, she said. She also noted that the summit is intended to be only the beginning of a call for change, and that attendees would be called upon to continue to collaborate and advance the issue in the weeks, months and years to come.

Trends and Perspectives

Brief summary: Three people – one employer representative, one physician and one nurse and researcher – shared their professional and personal insight into the issue of disability employment in the health care industry. For more background on each participant, please see Appendix B: Agenda.

Martha Artiles, Chief Diversity Officer, ManpowerGroup

ManpowerGroup has a long history of involvement in disability employment. As a workforce solution provider with 400,000 clients around the globe, it has significant insight into workforce trends and the skill sets corporations need to fill. As a result, it partners with governmental and non-government organizations to help them develop strategies for addressing current and projected labor shortages. Based on predicted trends, Manpower is currently paying particular attention to three populations: women, older workers and people with disabilities. Employers will need to figure out how to access these populations and increase their participation in the workforce in order to fulfill workforce needs in coming years, and the latter is perhaps most significant because it runs across all diverse segments. Furthermore, people with disabilities already exist in most organizations' workforces but may be unknown because they have chosen not to disclose.

Recently, ManpowerGroup partnered with the National Council on Disability to prepare a report titled *Workforce Infrastructure in Support of People with Disabilities: Matching Human Resources to Service Needs.* This report presents recommendations that call for partnerships among Federal departments and agencies, their state counterparts and the private sector, including education/training, health care and employment services organizations in order to overcome the projected shortfall in the disability services workforce and ensure continued gains in quality of life for people with disabilities. The report is divided into six sections, as follows:

1. Introduction and background
2. National trends, gaps and barriers, and their implications for people with disabilities and the disability services industry
3. Disability services infrastructure occupations: supply and demand
4. Private-sector strategies for building and maintaining a sufficient supply of disability infrastructure occupations
5. Public sector strategies for building and maintaining a sufficient supply of disability infrastructure occupations
6. Recommendations

For the report's executive summary, see Appendix C; *for the full report, visit* www.ncd.gov/publications/2010/Jan202010.

To monitor trends in employer needs, Manpower conducts an annual survey of about 40,000 employers worldwide. Even during the record-high unemployment of recent years, these surveys have consistently revealed that some jobs remain difficult to fill. In fact, the 2010 survey showed that 31 percent of employers said they were having difficulty filling all jobs, pointing to a talent mismatch in a variety of industries, one of which is health care. The top five jobs predicted to be most in demand in coming years—home health care aide (49 percent), medical assistant (35 percent), substance abuse counselor (34 percent), social and human services assistant (34 percent) and mental health counselor (30 percent)—are ones for which there is not enough talent in the pipeline.

Ensuring people with disabilities have access to education, health care and employment services is critical to meeting future workforce needs, and although positive trends are apparent, many barriers exist or have the potential to arise. *Workforce Infrastructure in Support of People with Disabilities: Matching Human Resources to Service Needs* provides recommendations to achieve this, five of which include:

- Establishing a mechanism to track, in real time, ongoing economic, social, labor market and professional developments so that new information can be used to redirect planning and actions in support of the disability services infrastructure;
- Gathering more definitive coverage regarding new and emerging jobs related to the disabilities service infrastructure, as tracked by the Bureau of Labor Statistics;
- Fully tapping people with disabilities, including Veterans with disabilities, through agency collaboration and ensuring accessible workplace environments;
- Forming effective private-public partnerships to fully fund and provide for the comprehensive range of social, educational and health care needs of all populations; and
- Creating systematic efforts, led by the National Institute on Disability and Rehabilitation Research (NIDRR) to acquire data from universities, training programs, professional organizations and unions on the supply of infrastructure workers, so that education and training resources can be realigned as needed to support the disability infrastructure workforce.

Stanley Yarnell, MD

Retired physician Dr. Yarnell started to lose his sight when he was 20 and was using a white stick by the time he was 38. During these years, he also trained for and developed a meaningful career as both a private practice physician and academic. As part of this, he had Stanford physical medicine and rehabilitation residents rotating with him at St. Mary's Hospital in San Francisco. One of these residents was Dr. Doug Ota, who acquired incomplete quadriplegia as a result of a diving accident when he was a junior in medical school. An experience working alongside Dr. Ota to assist a patient who suffered spine injuries and a traumatic brain injury in an automobile accident reinforced to Dr. Yarnell the unique position physicians with disabilities like he and Dr. Ota hold within the medical community.

Dr. Yarnell's self-identity as a person with a disability evolved over a number of years and really cemented when in 1984 he joined the board of the San Francisco Independent Living Resource Center, a step he took ostensibly out of concern for his patients, but also because of the camaraderie he felt with his fellow board members with disabilities.

In 1987, Dr. Yarnell's vision decreased sharply and he started using a white stick. Within a month of doing so, the administrator at the hospital where he was medical director of a small pediatric spinal cord injury rehabilitation unit asked him to step down for liability reasons. This resulted in shock, humiliation and anger, especially given that Dr. Yarnell was only just finding his emotional footing as a person and physician with a disability. Previously he felt that, given his expertise and experience, any good person would want to accommodate him.

This event occurred three years before the passage of the ADA, and the hospital wasn't subject to Section 504 of the Rehabilitation Act because it didn't receive Federal funds. While Dr. Yarnell's instinct was to let it go and focus on his private practice, he felt that if he was going to effectively advise his patients and advocate for their right to work, he also had to stand up for himself. He called upon the assistance of one of his patients, then Director of the Disability Rights Education and Defense Fund (DREDF), to seek recourse. The remedy that came out of this process that was most acceptable to him was a requirement that the hospital work with DREDF to develop policies to accommodate future employees with disabilities. At that point, Dr. Yarnell's identity as a person with a disability was firmly fixed, and he went on to join the boards of other related organizations, including the World Institute on Disability.

Drawing upon these experiences, Dr. Yarnell believes there are three key points that necessitate focus in order to improve educational and employment opportunities for people with disabilities in health care. Although clearly he sees these points in the context of his experience as a physician, he feels all three can be extrapolated to other health care occupations.

1) *The qualities that physicians with disabilities bring to the table for their patients and the institutions for which they work.* Dr. Yarnell's patients and their families valued his advice partly because of his own personal experience as a person with a disability. Furthermore, physicians without disabilities who work alongside physicians with disabilities often transform their own misconceptions, especially those of low expectations for workers with disabilities. Simple exposure breeds a higher level of comfort, acceptance and inclusion. Finally, physicians with disabilities are better able to scrutinize their own institutions and recognize needed improvements to better include both employees and patients with disabilities.

2) *Programs that may help physicians with disabilities in terms of career development.* Mentoring, informal networking and collaboration are key to career development for all people, but perhaps especially for medical professionals with disabilities. "Look-alike" mentoring programs should be encouraged so

that people training or new to the workforce can learn from others' experiences and strategies. Just before retirement, Dr. Yarnell was a preceptor and look-alike mentor for a blind medical student who subsequently graduated and completed his residency in psychiatry. This young doctor later told Dr. Yarnell that he learned more from him than his other preceptors, despite them also being very supportive. Brenda Primo, past Director of Rehabilitation for the State of California and current Director of the Office of Disabilities at Western University of Health Sciences, has been aggressive in setting up such mentorships, but they are not widely available at medical schools nationwide. Opportunities for networking among physicians with disabilities, including informal networking through the Internet, should also be encouraged. Staff support from organizations such as the American Medical Association, American Hospital Association and state medical associations, could help foster such opportunities.

3) *Manpower*. To achieve adequate representation of disability in positions of leadership in the medical community, there simply need to be more physicians with disabilities. This point was articulated well in a 2005 Journal of Physical Medicine and Rehabilitation article by Dr. Joel DeLisa that highlighted the very low percentage of people with disabilities in the physician workforce as compared to the general workforce, with the rate of medical students estimated at one percent. By Dr. Yarnell's informal estimates, this rate is even lower. Dr. DeLisa has put forth a number of recommendations to encourage students with disabilities to apply to and be admitted to medical school, one of which is revisiting goals and expectations for graduating students and residents to bring them in line with current technologies and ADA standards.

Beth Marks, RN, PhD

As President of the National Organization of Nurses with Disabilities, Beth Marks, along with Dr. Bronwynne Evans, produced a documentary film titled "Open the Door, Get 'Em a Locker: Educating Nursing Students with Disabilities," which chronicles the experiences of Victoria Christianson, who is believed to be the first student who uses a wheelchair to enter a four-year baccalaureate program in nursing. Dr. Evans was Victoria's clinical instructor. The film was released two years ago and offers insight into not only Victoria's trials and triumphs, but also the experiences of her peers, teachers and clinical preceptors. In doing so, it draws upon both the medical model and social model of disability to explore roles and responsibilities in nursing education.

A portion of the film "Open the Door, Get 'Em a Locker: Educating Nursing Students with Disabilities" was shown. Excerpts from the film, as well as information about how to obtain the full 23-minute version in DVD form, is available online at www.nurseswithdisabilities.org.

Panel I: The Clinical Setting: New Strategies

Brief summary: Five people representing a range of clinical health care professions, including physician, nurse and occupational therapist, shared their personal experiences and efforts to improve access to and employment in health care for people with disabilities. For more background on each participant, please see Appendix B: Agenda.

Kristi Kirschner, MD (Moderator)

Physician and medical professor Dr. Kirschner first became interested in the employment of people with disabilities in the health care field 20 years ago, when she worked alongside a fellow resident who had recently acquired quadriplegia. She and this colleague spent significant time brainstorming what he could and could not do and what he needed in terms of supports to finish his residency. Through this process, she found herself also contemplating the wealth of knowledge, clinical judgment and personal experience he would now bring his profession, something she witnessed this first hand later on when she had a young patient with a spinal cord injury. When she took this colleague to see the patient, the patient responded to him on a very different level, asking hard questions and seeking straight information from him versus her, who had only theoretical knowledge. Since this time, she has also learned a great deal from another peer with a disability.

Throughout her career, Dr. Kirschner has also observed with interest the experiences of medical students or potential medical students with disabilities. One of these was Jim Post, an outstanding undergraduate student with quadriplegia who was denied admission by ten medical schools despite very strong grades and admission test scores. Undeterred, he applied to nine schools the next year and was admitted to one, the Albert Einstein Medical School in New York. He went on to graduate in the top five percent of his class in 1997. Accommodations he needed to complete medical school included lower exam tables and the use of a physician's assistant for motor skills; he covered these at his own expense. He went on to complete his residency in internal medicine and a fellowship in nephrology and today is a nephrologist at a New York VA facility. In a recent article, Dr. Post commented that it would actually be harder for him to get into medical school today than it was in the 1990s because of tightened standards for motor skills physicians must be able to perform, standards attributed to medical licensing examinations.

Another example, that of Dr. Sam Sims, who acquired quadriplegia in 1999 after a car accident, also highlights this important issue. After significant despair over the perceived loss of his ability to practice medicine, Dr. Sims realized that the critical skills of an emergency room physician are primarily cognitive, and that for fine motor tasks he couldn't perform any longer, he could use a physician's assistant or nurse practitioner, a true representation of the concept of team medicine. After this epiphany, Dr. Sims convinced his employer to allow him a six-month probationary period during which a back-up doctor would always be available while he was on duty. He has remained in his position ever since. Thus, examining standards for technical motor and sensory skills is key to increasing representation of people with disabilities in health care occupations, especially in the age of team medicine; long gone are the days when lone practitioners were expected to do everything.

Bronwynne Evans, PhD, RN

Dr. Bronwynne Evans is a long-time advocate for the inclusion of people with disabilities in the nursing profession. She has significant experience working with vulnerable populations including the elderly, Latinos, Native Americans and people with disabilities, in both clinical and classroom settings. This unique set of experiences helps her understand disability through the lens of cultural diversity. Research shows that the best care is provided by culturally and linguistically congruent professionals. Therefore, it is essential to have a diverse nursing workforce in terms of not only ethnicity and culture, but also disability, and achieving this requires a change in attitudes and the removal of various programmatic, communication and physical barriers.

One major barrier is what has become known as "functional abilities," stemming from a study done in 1996 by Carolyn Yokom meant to focus on employment. According to their author, these functional abilities were never intended for use as admittance guidelines for nursing schools; however, many have adopted them as such, creating tremendous barriers to entry for people with disabilities. The National Council of State Boards of Nursing have removed them from its website in recent years, but many nursing schools have direct lifts of them in their admission information. Dr. Evans and others want the organization to go one step further and publicly state that such use is inappropriate.

As an alternative, she promotes the use of technical standards tailored for education, not employment, looking to Section 504 of the Rehabilitation Act for guidance because it permits such standards as long as they do not exclude people with disabilities and include information about accommodations. As an example, a poorly worded standard might state that a nursing student "must be able to talk to a patient." A better, non-exclusionary version would say a nursing student "must be able to communicate effectively with a patient using various means." Another example of a well-written standard is "gather vital signs using a variety of means," as opposed to "hear a murmur through a stethoscope." In other words, to be fair and equitable, the focus of the standard should be on the skill, not a physical ability or attribute. Furthermore, standards should not address something learned in a nursing program.

A 2010 report titled *The Future of Nursing: Leading Change, Advancing Health* conducted by the Robert Wood Johnson Foundation and the Institute of Medicine highlighted the role nurses can play in helping the U.S. get out of its current health care morass. One solution is third-party reimbursement for nurses who provide direct primary care for people, including people with disabilities. Models of care that use advanced practice nurses in leadership roles can help promote positive health outcomes and decrease costs.

Strategies for ensuring a future, highly skilled nursing workforce inclusive of people with disabilities include loan forgiveness for students with disabilities; hiring faculty with disabilities at salaries high enough to keep them in academia; funding incentives; demonstration projects; and recognition for schools that excel at admitting and supporting students with disabilities. Furthermore, state boards of nursing need to root out inappropriate use of functional abilities and instead, as addressed above, promote good technical standards.

Nursing education should hold students to their theoretical knowledge and recognize that students remember their own self-regulation needs; students and nurses with disabilities aren't going to practice in environments where they are unsafe and unsure. Nursing is about much more than skills that can be taught to many people, such as CPR and drawing blood. Furthermore, nursing education needs disability content integrated into curricula.

Nurses' intellectual contributions to health care are sometimes overlooked, despite many being competent scholars as well as compassionate care providers. They must have a seat at the table to address the predicted increase in demand for their skills and knowledge. Better data across the profession is needed in order to effectively plan because nurses, including those with disabilities, are an invaluable resource in the effort to reform the nation's health care system.

Sandy Hanebrink, OTR/L

Sandy Hanebrink has a distinguished career spanning many roles, including a school system occupational therapist; clinical researcher; social security administration disability program expert; ADA, accessibility and assistive technology consultant; and non-profit director. In addition, she is a former Paralympic athlete and disabled sports coordinator. Her main interest is in education and employment issues, in particular promoting the inclusion of people with disabilities, like herself, in the occupational therapy profession.

Ms. Hanebrink developed quadriplegia in her early 20s as a result of an allergic reaction to medicine. Previously, she was a collegiate and Olympic hopeful athlete. During rehabilitation, she was referred to a disabled sports program and shortly thereafter became the assistant director. During this time, based on her skills and interests, several of her health care professionals suggested that she consider a career in sports medicine or occupational therapy. At first she had difficulty envisioning how doing so would be possible, but eventually she successfully navigated government programs in place to help people with disabilities pursue their career goals. She applied to an occupational therapy program in South Carolina without disclosing her disability and was accepted.

Once enrolled, the most challenging barriers Ms. Hanebrink faced were more attitudinal than architectural (although there were many of those too). For example, her fieldwork coordinator was of the mindset that she — not Ms. Hanebrink — should decide what Ms. Hanebrink's limitations and needs were. Furthermore, Ms. Hanebrink discovered that the program was, unbeknownst to her, disclosing information about her disability to fieldwork sites. In her current work as chair of a network of practitioners with disabilities and supports in the occupational therapy field, she has discovered that such discriminatory practices are still commonplace today, a paradox given the profession's supposed purpose to help people do what they want in life.

Today, Ms. Hanebrink works to get policies in place at the national level, through American Occupational Therapy Association (AOTA); however, doing so has proven to be a slow process. Again, many of the barriers are attitudinal and many have to do with misunderstanding of what makes someone a good occupational therapist. For example, some express concern about how an occupational therapist with a disability might physically transfer someone, not recognizing that the most important ability an occupational therapist offers is intellectual; an occupational therapist teaches. But misconceptions still stem from the medical model in which a disability is viewed as something needing to be fixed. There needs to be a shift in thinking to a social model in which, once barriers are removed, everyone is equal and disability is just another form of diversity. However, within the profession, disability is not incorporated into talk about the need for a culturally competent and diverse workforce, and AOTA, the national voice for the profession, does not currently collect relevant data or provide sufficient support to advance the cause.

Rosemary Ciotti, RN, MSN, CRNP

Rosemary Ciotti is president of Accessible Living, Inc. in Arlington, Virginia, through which she works primarily with persons with spinal cord injuries. The company's guiding philosophy is "to live well with a disability requires accessible housing, education, employment, transportation and health care." In addition to her clinical practice, she chairs the Arlington County Planning Commission, working to make Arlington a more accessible community.

Ms. Ciotti acquired her disability well into a distinguished career as a nurse and educator. Previously, she was at the University of Pennsylvania, where she worked alongside a perinatologist and ran a high-volume clinic for underserved women. In the 1980s, she also ran a clinic for underserved women in New Jersey, where she saw dreadful health conditions resulting from lack of access to effective prevention and treatment services; some patients had never even seen physicians. Patients did not have insurance, and often their immigration status was suspect, but Ms. Ciotti was committed to soliciting funds to care for this population because of her strong belief that health care is a human right and should not be tied to whether someone could hold a job or had the right papers.

Around this time, Ms. Ciotti developed problems walking and starting having chest pain. She was diagnosed with a range of conditions and developed quadriplegia as a result of them. Expectations that she would live were low. She was sent to hospice, but "failed" it, defying her doctors' predictions. She then began the journey of learning to live with a disability. Her community had no accessibility infrastructure, and her only association of disability was with the elderly, not those of working age. Eventually, her husband accepted a job in Washington, D.C., and they moved to nearby Arlington, Virginia, which had more of an accessibility infrastructure in place, partly due to the metropolitan area's Metro system. They also found accessible housing suitable for their family, which at that time included a baby and two grade-school children.

However, it was still some time until Ms. Ciotti found that she could live well. Her speech was significantly impaired, something that took occupational therapy and two years of hard work to improve. In addition, she felt trapped, and came to understand the importance of the built environment in living well as a person with a disability. Lack of accessibility impeded her ability to take care of her children and herself and impacted her mental health.

As time went on, Ms. Ciotti recovered and started to meet more and more non-elderly people with disabilities living and working in the D.C. area, many focused on issues related to disability such as transportation or housing. But she found that little attention was being paid to health care — something that also needs to be accessible to live well. Given her professional background, she found herself starting to fill this gap, providing preventative screenings and health care services for people with disabilities. Many of these people, unlike the ones she worked with in New Jersey, had health insurance; they simply couldn't use it because facilities were often inaccessible, despite many being required to be so under Federal regulations, including the Rehabilitation Act of 1973.

Eventually, Ms. Ciotti felt ready to seek employment, but could not find a job. Having worked in some capacity since she was 13 and amassed significant clinical experience and expertise, this was a demoralizing experience. After some of the people with disabilities she had become acquainted with started coming to her with health care-related concerns, she realized that her skills were very much needed within the disability community. From this, her career was reborn. Her patients lived in wheelchair accessible apartments and had attendants to assist them, and perhaps most important, related to her in a way they might not other providers. Patients' doctors responded positively to her services because often they were unable to adequately serve these patients due to accessibility issues. This caused many patients to end up in the emergency room or intensive care unit because they stayed home until problems became urgent. Preventative care and access to services for all people, including people with disabilities, is key to ensuring health care reform works.

There is a need for greater understanding and education within nursing and medical community at large about the value and qualities practitioners with disabilities bring to the field. This is central to the mission of the National Organization of Nurses with Disabilities, which Ms. Ciotti is active in along with Beth Marks, Bronwynne Evans, Karen McCulloh and others. Anecdotal evidence suggests that significant problems occur relative to the care of people with disabilities because of a simple lack of understanding. There is a smarter way to deliver health care, particularly to people with disabilities, and nurses and other health care professionals with disabilities have an important role to play in doing so, especially during this important time of health care reform.

Susan Douglas, MD, JD

Dr. Douglas is a physician who today works as a public policy consultant and independent advisor on the Affordable Care Act. The daughter of a doctor and nurse, she found herself naturally inclined toward a health care career. Growing up in that environment, she also learned about the power of exposure in overcoming prejudice. Her family was the only biracial family in her community, and when medical care was needed, her father's availability as a doctor sometimes forced some people to rise above their biases. She feels this lesson has relevance to misconceptions about disability and employment.

Six months into medical school, Dr. Douglas sustained a spinal cord injury in a car accident. When she returned, the school didn't exactly know how to accommodate her, and she didn't always know what she needed either. No one in a wheelchair had attended the school previously. However, the year she graduated, the school admitted another individual who uses a wheelchair.

The first two years of medical school are primarily classroom-based, and during this time she didn't encounter many problems aside from physical barriers. Some of these barriers were easily accommodated; others required her to request assistance, something she was often reluctant to do because of the highly competitive nature of medical school. It would have been better if there had been a system in place to help her anticipate her needs.

The clinical years were more problematic because they required Dr. Douglas to navigate hospital facilities, something daunting to many doctors in training regardless of disability. Fortunately, her first rotation was in neurology, where she found that she had a different relationship with patients than other students. Her chairman noticed this and took her under his wing. A particularly compelling moment came when she assisted a patient who had suffered a bad stroke in being able to relax and breathe through a ventilator by sharing her personal experience of having had to do so. She didn't encounter as supportive an environment in her other rotations, particularly surgery, where the chairman actually commented negatively about her prospects for being a surgeon. In hindsight she wishes she had challenged him on his bias.

After completing medical school and practicing at UCLA, she joined the faculty but, through her experience as both a physician and patient, became increasingly frustrated with the bureaucratic side of heath care. She felt the focus was in the wrong place, and that insurance companies were the problem. So, she went to law school and completed a public policy fellowship on Capitol Hill. This experience reinforced to her even more how critical it is for people with disabilities to have a seat at the table in the policymaking process, something she now works to achieve in her daily work.

Panel I – Questions and Discussion

Participants posed the following questions or comments following Panel I:

- A psychologist said that in addition to the stories she heard during the panel, she'd like to hear more about health care professionals who are deaf or hard of hearing. The ability to communicate effectively is a critical skill, and there are only 20 known deaf doctors in the U.S. Gallaudet University, Rochester Institute of Technology's National Technical Institute for the Deaf and other organizations have started a task force to figure out how to improve the representation of the deaf community in health care professions. Changing technical standards into functional standards, as discussed by several speakers, is essential to doing so.

- o Dr. Douglas remarked that it's important that it be viewed as a civil rights issue while at the same time considering quality in standards. Ms. Hanebrink said that the key is not just getting policies in place, but ensuring they are enforced. Ms. Ciotti echoed this, noting that hospitals may be willing to hire but still may not have facilities in compliance with Federal requirements, so people can't actually work.

- A registered nurse said that when she first started to look into nursing, she was told by a community college that she could not work in the profession because she would not be able to navigate a hospital in a wheelchair. Thomas Jefferson University in Philadelphia did welcome her; however, she was told she could not use her wheelchair in hospital rooms. At the time, she didn't know there was a problem with that stipulation. She worked without her wheelchair, but with pain and discomfort, because she felt she needed to go above and beyond to prove herself. However, she has not been able to get a job in a hospital. Coming together with other health care professionals with disabilities at the summit has helped her learn that she is not alone, and she is eager to advocate, educate and work to change attitudes going forward.

- A physician with a disability said this summit is the best conference she's attended and then shared her story of having attended medical school, completed a fellowship and established a career with a disability, working for a long time until her symptoms became devastating. Her disability took away her identity and displaced her. She's pleased to hear the stories of other women like her because it helps her see her place amongst their community and that she still has significant value to add.

- Dr. Kirschner asked panel members why they felt, given the huge advances in technology in recent years, things appear to be getting worse, not better relative to access to employment in health care for people with disabilities.

- o Ms. Hanebrink said she often asks her colleagues the same thing, and that she feels much of it has to do with attitudinal barriers, health care culture and lack of regulatory enforcement at the Federal level. She said practitioners in her field with nonvisible disabilities also face significant barriers because of misconceptions and stereotypes.

- o Dr. Douglas said a problem she saw when she was on the UCLA admissions committee is the rite of passage culture, that doctors feel that medical students must go through the same experiences despite technological changes and advances that can open doors for people with disabilities.

- o Dr. Evans said a similar tradition-bound culture exists in nursing and that, particularly in nursing education, there is a lack of awareness that this is a civil rights issue, something particularly ironic given nurses' mission to help people. Aggressive measures need to be taken regarding compliance and in incorporating disability into curricula. But to do so, help from higher up is needed, because the National Organization of Nurses with Disabilities is an all-volunteer force without a lot of power or money.

- A psychologist asked whether there is data about how much employers' fear of liability factors into these discriminatory practices. Panelists generally agreed that they have heard anecdotally that it's a real issue, that doctors with disabilities who are trying to get jobs frequently get asked questions about liability. Dr. Douglas said that in cases where she has served as an expert witness, no one could cite a single incident to support doctors with disabilities being a liability; however, the perception that they are is the reality with insurance companies.

- Dr. Yarnell said activities such as publishing in professional journals can help raise awareness of the issue among health care professionals and mentioned specifically an upcoming article by Dr. DeLisa about the ADA Amendments Act and its implications for residency and medical school.

- Dr. Kirschner closed the session by noting to Assistant Secretary Martinez that panelists' stories all echo a need for more success stories about people with a range of disabilities in the health care field and for concrete, practical suggestions about accommodations, including in the educational environment.

Luncheon Speaker

Patricia A. Shiu, Director, Office of Federal Contract Compliance Programs (OFCCP), U.S. Department of Labor

Ms. Shiu began by thanking Assistant Secretary Martinez, Access Living and summit organizers for inviting her to speak. She also recognized her special assistant Claudia Gordon and expressed appreciation to Kareem Dale for his guidance and insight during the process of revising OFCCP's Section 503 regulations, which require Federal contractors to take affirmative action to hire and advance in employment people with disabilities.

At a recent civil rights dinner honoring Hubert Humphrey, Ms. Shiu was reminded that he once remarked that the moral test of government is how it treats those at the start of life, the end of life and in the shadows of life. She affirmed to summit participants that today's administration believes that no one should be relegated to the shadows; Secretary Solis and President Obama see people with disabilities, as do Assistant Secretary Martinez and herself, and people with disabilities are included in the President's call to "win the future."

When Ms. Shiu and her colleagues arrived in 2009, things were in disarray from years of neglect. However, great strides have been made, for example, the signing of the Christopher and Dana Reeve Paralysis Act; United Nations Convention on the Rights of Persons with Disabilities; Executive Order 13548 (Increasing Federal Employment of Individuals with Disabilities); and the 21st Century Communications and Video Accessibility Act. Furthermore, EEOC just published final regulations implementing the ADA Amendments Act of 2008.

OFCCP's job is to hold those who do business with the Federal government accountable to the fair and reasonable obligation to take affirmative action and not discriminate in employment on the basis of race/ethnicity, disability or status as a Veteran. Its scope is wide; nearly one in four workers in America is employed by a Federal contractor or subcontractor, and a large number of companies in the health care industry fall under OFCCP's jurisdiction.

OFCCP audits about 4,000 companies randomly each year. It also supports the good faith work of employers, especially small business employers, who want to do the right thing. But for those employers who refuse, OFCCP is aggressive about enforcement. Being a Federal contractor is a privilege, not a right, and with that privilege comes obligations. OFCCP forces violators to correct bad policies. It also helps victims. Those who don't want to follow the law will not get contracts.

Currently, OFCCP is in the most important period of regulatory reform in its history, working to update its laws to reflect today's workplaces. One of these laws is Section 503 of the Rehabilitation Act. Despite this law being on the books for nearly 30 years, the employment rate disparity between people with disabilities and people without disabilities remains unacceptable. So, last year OFCCP worked closely with ODEP to issue an Advance Notice of Proposed Rulemaking (ANPRM) seeking input into how to strengthen it, and in a few months will be issuing a Notice of Proposed Rulemaking (NPRM) seeking additional comments from the public. The revising of Section 503 will be historic, and Ms. Shiu is committed to not just implementation, but also strong enforcement.

Ms. Shiu's dedication to this issue stems from her long career as a civil rights attorney in San Francisco. In this role, she learned that work is about much more than a paycheck; it's about dignity and self-respect. When the ADA was passed in 1990, she hoped it would serve as the floor for good practices, not the ceiling, and this hope drove her to represent numerous people with disabilities in fighting for their rights in employment, education and community life. In leading OFCCP, she strives to further advance this spirit, to raise expectations, not lower them, in support of Secretary Solis's vision of good jobs for everyone.

Participants posed the following questions or comments following Ms. Shiu's presentation:

- A participant asked for a timeline for release of the Section 503 NPRM. Ms. Shiu said it is in its last stages and going to the Office of Management and Budget (OMB) shortly. Of the regulations OFCCP is working on, this was the most intellectually difficult one, she said, noting that ODEP was a critical partner in developing sensible and enforceable proposed regulations. In addition, she remarked that currently, when OFCCP audits a company, it checks for accessibility and policies related to disability, whether or not there is a Section 503 claim, in order to help make clear what is expected of employers.

- A participant asked about the number of contractors whose contracts have been revoked under OFCCP regulations. Ms. Shiu replied that in the history of OFCCP, it's only been a handful, because such action isn't what's desired since it would put people out of jobs. Rather, revocation is the very last sanction after all else has failed. But, there are currently three cases pending (University of Pittsburgh Medical Center, Bank of America and United Space Alliance), she said, noting that these companies didn't necessarily violate the law but rather refused to provide required data, which is OFCCP's "lifeblood."

Panel II: Career Opportunities: Growth in Demand

Brief summary: Four people representing employer networks and unions shared their involvement in efforts to improve access to and employment in health care for people with disabilities, in both clinical and non-clinical settings. For more background on each participant, please see Appendix B: Agenda.

Brigida Hernandez, PhD (Moderator)

Dr. Hernandez is Director of Research for the YAI Network, an alliance of non-profit health and human services agencies that serve people of all ages with disabilities New York City. She is also a researcher, and when she was at DePaul University collaborated with several other organizations on a three-year study titled *Exploring the Bottom Line: The Costs and Benefits of Workers with Disabilities in the Health Care Sector*. This study had two phases, the first qualitative and the second quantitative.

Study 1 consisted of a focus group with 12 administrators from seven large hospitals in the Chicago area. These focus groups revealed the following themes:

1. Disability employment agencies and champions were critical for recruiting, hiring and building corporate culture;
2. Frontline managers were viewed as having biases and concerns with job performance and costs;
3. Promotion opportunities were limited, with many holding semi-skilled positions (clerical, food service, laundry);
4. Costs were viewed as minimal and worth the expense; and
5. Benefits included dedicated and reliable employees and a diverse workforce.

Study 2 gathered data from eight Chicago area hospitals to compare the work-related variables (i.e., tenure, absenteeism, job performance, supervision, workers' compensation claims and accommodations) of workers with and without disabilities. Results indicated that workers with disabilities had similar ratings for job performance and amount of supervision required. Documented accommodation requests and costs were minimal (an average of $521, which comports with cost data analyzed by the Job Accommodation Network (JAN) across all industries).

Areas where workers with disabilities did not fare as well as counterparts without disabilities were tenure, unscheduled absences and, to a lesser degree, the number of workers' compensation claims. However, it is important to note that this was a first attempt to gather this sort of information and from a limited geographical area, therefore, generalizations should be made with caution. *For a more extensive summary of the report's findings, see Appendix D.*

Kevin Shanklin, MBA

Kevin Shanklin is Executive Director in the Office of the President and CEO of Blue Cross Blue Shield (BCBS) Association in Chicago. His company insures hundreds of millions of Americans through 39 member plans. As one of the group health plan options Federal employees have, BCBS is also a Federal contractor. Although the insurance industry is often perceived as a barrier to improving access to health care, Mr. Shanklin and the people he works with on a daily basis are dedicated to collaborating and being a part of the solution to problems with the nation's health care system.

In fact, BCBS recognizes that the Affordable Care Act presents an opportunity. Because of it, many people will be entering the insurance market for the first time, and it's likely many of these will be people with disabilities because this population has a lower rate of employment, and insurance has historically been linked to employment. This represents a fundamental shift in the way BCBS operates, moving away from a business-to-business model through which it had to sell itself to one person—a benefits manager—and toward a business-to-individual model through which it has to sell itself to one person at a time.

Furthermore, BCBS is committed to not only serving people with disabilities as members, but also ensuring they are represented in its workforce. Two member plan examples exemplify this commitment: BCBS of Florida and BCBS of Massachusetts.

BCBS of Florida takes an active leadership role in Florida's Business Leadership Network (BLN), and in partnership with the University of North Florida and the Governor's Office, received $75,000 to create a series of internships for students with disabilities with BLN member companies across Florida. Internships are six to eight weeks in length and paid at a rate of $10-12 per hour. Thus far, the program has resulted in a 35 percent post-internship employment rate.

BCBS of Florida also has an internal program through its Employee Resource Group (ERG), called "PosAbilities." This ERG is heavily involved in BCBS of Florida's diversity initiatives and look at disability across various aspects of BCBS of Florida's business operations, not just employment, but also suppliers and customers. It also established nearly 50 internships within the company and coordinated BCBS of Florida's involvement in Disability Mentoring Day (DMD).

BCBS of Massachusetts is also working with students with disabilities as a way to promote positive future employment outcomes. The organization had a two-day employment event that convened 60 recent college graduates with disabilities from across New England as well as New York. One day of this event was dedicated to interview sessions with major employers.

Providing opportunities to gain on-the-job experience through internships is a critical aspect of these programs. In fact, an internship is what propelled Mr. Shanklin to his ongoing, highly rewarding career. As a young person, he was provided such an opportunity through an organization called INROADS, which then and today works to introduce minority students to business careers through multi-year internships. He has been with BCBS for 30 years and is proud to spend his time working on ways to improve how millions of Americans interact with the health care system. An internship and open-minded workplace culture is what got him started, and he is committed paying it forward for others, including young people with disabilities.

Yvette Crespo

Yvette Crespo is Director of Recruitment Operations at Kaiser Permanente, one of the largest non-profit health plans in the nation. Founded in 1945, the company today serves several regions and has a total of 35 hospitals and additional 454 medical offices. It has about 15,000 partner physicians and 165,000 employees. Ms. Crespo takes great pride in her job and Kaiser's organizational culture, which one of her projects, Project SEARCH, exemplifies. When she first floated the idea of PROJECT Search, a work-experience program for transitioning high school students with disabilities, Ms. Crespo encountered ambivalence from managers. But she and a colleague persevered and implemented a pilot in 2008 with the help of service agencies, including vocational rehabilitation. Now, there are several new sites, and her vision is to have a program in place at every Kaiser facility by 2014. To date, about 50 interns have completed six-week internships providing skills training for entry-level positions within Kaiser facilities.

As part of Kaiser's commitment to ensuring its workforce reflects the communities it serves, the organization is also working to update its materials to include "unconscious bias" training for hiring managers and employees and focusing on obtaining contracts from diverse vendors, including disability-owned businesses.

Based on Ms. Crespo's experience with Project SEACH and other initiatives, she feels that in order to make significant progress, young people with disabilities must have the opportunity to learn, through first-hand experience, the value they have to offer organizations and the important role competitive employment plays in transitioning to adulthood and independence. Likewise, employers need to learn how people with disabilities can help fill needed skill sets and better serve and reflect their customer base.

To achieve this, Ms. Crespo would like the U.S. Department of Labor and other organizations to offer more funding for training programs geared toward competitive employment. Exposure, options and training are key to driving real change. By offering these, Kaiser has learned the value people with disabilities have to offer, not just through practical job skills, but also motivation, commitment and work ethic — the essential employee attributes that build strong organizations and communities.

The Project SEARCH program started at Cincinnati Children's Hospital Medical Center in 1996 and today has grown to more than 150 programs, including Kaiser's. For more information about the Project SEARCH model, visit www.projectsearch.us.

David Mulvey, MSW

David Mulvey is a Service Coordinator at California's Tri-Counties Regional Center and since 1997 has also chaired the Service Employee International Union's (SEIU) California Committee on Developmental Disabilities. As part of this position, he worked in collaboration with several organizations, including the World Institute on Disability, to get SEIU to pass resolution 119a, titled "SEIU has Good Things for Persons with Disabilities." Adopted in 2008, this resolution was designed as a tool to develop partnerships to create good union jobs for people with disabilities.

One way unions can support work for people with disabilities is to protect them and their rights under laws such as the FMLA and ADA through training for staff and members. Another strategy is to partner with unions on their existing training programs. One example is an educational partnership between the Los Angeles Health Care system, country workforce development services and Mr. Mulvey's union local. This partnership offers low-wage employees an opportunity to upgrade their skills in order to obtain health care jobs in Los Angeles County and takes pride in supporting non-traditional learners. While it hasn't specifically targeted people with disabilities, it stands ready to do so. Employers can go to locals and work with them through programs such as this to learn how to accommodate workers with disabilities in training programs.

SEIU has also worked to advance disability employment through its involvement in passage of Proposition 63, the Mental Health Services Act in California. In addition to bringing in new revenue to mental health services in California, this proposition provides for employment and training of people who received mental health services as peer counselors. Following its passage, one of the people who helped author this resolution, himself a parent of a son with autism, met with the director of East Bay Innovations, which provides vocational and independent living supports for people with developmental disabilities, to discuss how to act on it. They put together a grant proposal, funded by the local, to bring in job development experts from Washington State who conducted joint training for SEIU members from San Francisco and Easy Bay Innovations on how to effectively get people with disabilities on the job in union environments.

SEIU and SEIU employers have also benefitted from Project SEARCH, as evidenced through the experiences of two students, Derek and Joel. Derek, a person with a development disability, had worked in a Regional Occupational Program (ROP)-funded job in a local hospital in high school, but was told after graduation that there were no paid positions. He then participated in Project SEARCH at Children's Hospital in Oakland and did well, but continued to talk with his job coach about wanting to go back to his local hospital.

So, the job coach talked to his ROP teacher and met with his previous manager at the hospital, who said he'd like to hire him but couldn't because the workforce was unionized and there were no unionized classifications he met. The job coach, who had received training and was aware of Resolution 119a, went to the local and they crafted an agreement that set aside a position for persons with developmental disabilities that would not supplant existing staff. In turn, the union agreed that the position would be exempt from normal layoffs. Today, Derek is a proud union member earning $14.58 per hour. He is thriving and makes the hospital a better place, for workers and patients.

SEIU also worked with East Bay Innovations to establish a Project SEARCH site in county government, which had never done before. Joel, a young man with autism, was in the first class. Despite a high level of intelligence and a college degree, Joel had not been successful in employment due to social skills deficits. His first Project SEARCH rotation was in the Sheriff's Department Human Resources office, where the manager asked Joel to assist with clearing a backlog of cases, a task expected to take a few weeks. Joel finished in one day. When it came time for Joel to move to his next rotation, the manager asked if he could stay. Project SEARCH mangers said sure – if he was hired as a paid employee. However, civil service rules created a barrier. But, Joel's job coach informed the manager about Step-Up, which sets aside positions for workers with disabilities in the county outside of civil service requirements. Today, Joel is a county employee and union member making $39,000 a year – more than his job coach.

These are just a few examples of how organizations can partner with SEIU to improve employment opportunities for people with disabilities. Mr. Mulvey encouraged summit participants to contact their local SEIU representatives to learn more.

Panel II – Questions and Discussion

Participants posed the following questions or comments following Panel II:

- A participant commented that one problem she has seen is that sometimes, even after phenomenal internships programs through which students work for multiple summers, there is no job waiting for them upon graduation. This not only provides false hopes, but also is inefficient cost-wise on the part of the organization, because all the money spent training these individuals ends up ultimately benefitting another organization.
- A participant asked Dr. Hernandez if anyone has duplicated her research.
  - Dr. Hernandez replied that the closest duplication was a similar cost-benefit study conducted in Australia. However, a big difference was that individuals in the Australia study had self-disclosed their

disability, while the DePaul study included both people who had disclosed and people who had not. Furthermore, the Australian study was not industry specific. The DePaul study looked at a few industries, not just health care. There are also many studies that look at employer attitudes regarding the employment of people with disabilities, but typically they have measured perceptions, not hard data.

- A participant asked Dr. Hernandez why tenure measured shorter among people with disabilities in her study.
  - o Dr. Hernandez replied that because the information about tenure was strictly quantitative and only gathered at one point in time, conclusions could not be drawn or generalizations made. More data, over more time, is needed.
- Beverly Huckman, Associate VP for Equal Opportunity Rush University Medical College and Chair, Rush's ADA Task Force said she feels the key to advancing disability employment lies in corporate culture and commitment, things that take work, but not a lot of money, to change. Key is support from the very top and reflecting this, Rush's ADA task force includes strong representation from upper management. Because of this, if the taskforce puts a program forth, it is automatically perceived as important, regardless of whether it's a budget line item. This critical value of high-level commitment in making disability part of organizational culture is supported by research.
- Alan Muir, Executive Director, Career Opportunities for Students with Disabilities remarked that his group collaborated with BCBS of Massachusetts on the event about which Kevin Shanklin talked. As a result of this event, Microsoft "bought one student directly off of the showroom floor" and not long after, he became a full-time employee. A similar summit was held at Cisco Systems in San Jose, California, where Cisco and NBC Universal both hired students. He hopes to have an event in Chicago next year. His organization also has an annual event in New Jersey.

Karen McCulloh, RN, BS

Karen McCulloh served as the subject matter expert for the summit and appreciates greatly everyone's contributions to the dialogue and hopes lessons learned will now be carried nationwide throughout the health care industry, because great care was taken to ensure diversity among participants, both in terms of occupation and geographical representation.

Ms. McCulloh is a working nurse who is in the deaf/blind category and co-founded the National Organization of Nurses with Disabilities. She represents another example of sentiments expressed throughout the day, especially the early panels, that when you acquire a disability later in life, it's a big adjustment.

The day's discussions reveal a lot of work needs to be done. Just a few of the key themes emerging include:

- The need for more research into cultural competencies that people with disabilities bring to their job.
- Guidance on accommodations for employees and students with disabilities training for careers in health care, especially those who want to work "on the floor." Because of misconceptions about what people with disabilities can do, managers need to be better educated and equipped with information about accommodation resources.
- Technical standards need to be scrutinized; in some cases, they are actually against the law. Support from high-level government officials could help in achieving this.

Closing

Assistant Secretary Martinez ended the session by emphasizing that the day's discussions are meant to be merely a start to the conversation about how to improve employment and training opportunities for people with disabilities in health care. Participants will now be asked to continue contributing their knowledge and experience in order to assist ODEP in promoting effective policy in this area. A fully accessible online workspace, called ePolicyWorks Health Care, is available to facilitate ongoing collaboration, and all participants will be receiving information about how to access it soon.

Assistant Secretary Martinez also reiterated that the summit was the second in a series of such "sector summits," the first of which focused on entertainment and media. Related to this, she closed by showing a public service announcement titled "I Can," which was created by the ODEP-funded Campaign for Disability Employment (CDE), a collaborative of several leading disability and business organizations that works to raise awareness of the skills and talents of people with disabilities, in all industries.

Featuring seven people with disabilities sharing what they "can do" in the workplace when given the opportunity, "I Can" works to challenge misconceptions and elevate expectations about disability employment, and it has earned significant donated media time since its release early last year. It is available online at www.whatcanyoudocampaign.org, along with accompanying discussion guides and other materials that can assist organizations in furthering its important message that at work, it's what people can do that matters—a message echoed throughout the summit's discussions.

Appendix A: Participant List

Health Care: Career Trends, Best Practices & Call-to-Action Summit
Tuesday, May 17, 2011
Access Living of Metropolitan Chicago

Participant List

- **Alan Muir,** Executive Director, Career Opportunities for Students with Disabilities
- **Aletha Ottlinger,** Director, Human Resources, Resurrection Health Care
- **Amber Smock,** Director of Advocacy, Access Living (VIP Reception Only)
- **Anne Hirsh,** Project Manager, Job Accommodation Network
- **Araceli Gonzalez,** General Summit Registration Volunteer, Access Living
- **Barbara Otto,** CEO, Business Development Specialist
- **Bechara Chouchair,** Commissioner, Chicago Department of Public Health (VIP Reception Only)
- **Beth Marks, RN, PhD,** President, National Organization of Nurses with Disabilities
- **Beverly Huckman,** Associate VP for Equal Opportunity Rush University Medical College; Chair, Rush ADA Task Force
- **Bill Sinwell,** Disability Services Specialist, IL Department of Commerce & Economic Opportunity
- **Bill Tapp,** National Director, College of Direct Support
- **Brigida Hernandez, PhD,** Director of Research, YAI Network
- **Bronwynne Evans, PhD, RN, CNS, FNGNA,** First Vice President, National Organization of Nurses with Disabilities
- **Carol Abnathy,** National Health & Wellness Manager, Job Corps
- **Carolyn Jones,** Assistant Commissioner, City of Chicago, Mayor's Office for People With Disabilities
- **Claudia Gordon,** Special Assistant to the Director, DOL/OFCCP
- **Cheryl Potts,** Employment Project Manager, Chicago House
- **Chuck Conaty,** Business Development Specialist, DOL/ODEP
- **Colet Mitchell,** DOL/ODEP Employer Policy Team
- **Daisy Feidt,** Executive VP, Access Living
- **David Mulvey,** Service Coordinator, SEIU, TriCounties Regional Center
- **David Newburger,** Consultant, Starkloff Disability Institute
- **Debra A. Naddeo, BSN, RN,** Recent Graduate, Nursing Student
- **Diane Collins, MD,** Physician
- **Donna Zondlo,** Consultant, HCSC Senior Diversity & Inclusion
- **Douglas Morton,** Rehabilitative Services, IL Department of Human Services
- **Emilia Pablo-Montano,** Press Staff for Secretary of Labor Hilda L. Solis, (VIP Reception Only)
- **Eric Grossman,** Chairman, Access Living
- **Gary Arnold,** PR Coordinator, Access Living
- **Hope Adler,** Concepts, Inc.

- **Irene W. Leigh, PhD**, Co-Chair, Task Force on Healthcare Careers for People who are Deaf or Hard-Of-Hearing, Professor, Clinical Psychology Doctoral Program; Chair, Department of Psychology, Gallaudet University
- **Ivy McKinley,** Director, Human Resources, Our Lady of Resurrection Medical Center
- **Jean Ashmore,** President, Association of Higher Education & Disability (AHEAD)
- **Jean Morrell,** Consultant
- **Jeanne Regnante,** Chief of Staff, Office of Chief Medical Officer, Merck
- **Jim Ace,** Researcher, SEIU
- **Jen Haggard,** SEIU
- **Jerry Rauman,** CFO, Access Living (VIP Reception Only)
- **Joel H. Delofsky,** Coordinator, DOL/Veterans' Employment & Training Service (VETS) Jobs for Veterans Lead Center
- **Joyce Lane,** Board Member, OT Professor, Access Living
- **Juanita Irizarry,** Program Officer, Chicago Community Trust
- **Judy Panko Reis,** Healthcare Access Policy Analyst, Access Living
- **Judy Perloff,** Program Director, Chicago House
- **Judy Reinhold,** President, Kaliber Imaging, Inc.
- **Judy Young,** National Employer Technical Assistance Center, Cornell University
- **Julie Carroll,** Senior Attorney/Advisor, National Council on Disability
- **Kareem Dale,** Associate Director, White House Office of Public Engagement & Special Assistant to the President for Disability Policy, The White House
- **Karen McCulloh,** President & CEO, Karen McCulloh & Associates Consulting
- **Karen Quammen,** National Project SEARCH Consultant, Project SEARCH
- **Karen Steffan,** LADSE Vocational Alliance
- **Karen Tamley,** Commissioner, City of Chicago, Mayor's Office for People with Disabilities
- **Kathleen Galvin,** HR Director, Rehabilitation Institute of Chicago
- **Kathleen Wilson-Thompson,** SVP of Human Resources, Walgreen Co.
- **Ken Skord,** Director, Vocational Services, Marianjoy Rehab Hospital
- **Kevin Scanlan,** President/CEO, Metropolitan Chicago Healthcare Council (MCHC) (VIP Reception Only)
- **Kevin Shanklin,** Executive Director, Office of the President, Blue Cross Blue Shield
- **Kimberly Wilson,** General Summit Registration Volunteer, Access Living
- **Kris Balfanz-Vertiz,** Coordinator, Extended Services Program, Deaf Access Program, Schwab Rehabilitation Hospital
- **Kristi Kirschner, MD,** Physical Medicine & Rehabilitation, Schwab Physician's Group, Schwab Rehabilitation Hospital
- **Dr. Larry Goodman,** CEO, Rush Medical Center
- **Linda B. Roberts, MSN, RN,** Manager, Illinois Center for Nursing, IL Department of Financial & Professional Regulation, Division of Professional Regulation
- **Lisa Braganca,** Legal Director, Access Living (VIP Reception Only)
- **Lisa Wiemken,** VIP Reception Registration Volunteer, Access Living
- **Loretta Herrington,** Partner, EIN SOF Communications
- **Lynnae Ruttledge,** Rehabilitation Services Administration (RSA) Commissioner, U.S. Department of Education

- **Maria Flynn,** Vice President, Jobs for the Future
- **Maria Heidkamp,** Senior Research Project Manager, John J. Heldrich Center for Workforce Development
- **Mark Williams,** Director, DisabilityWorks
- **Martha Artiles,** Chief Diversity Officer, ManPower Inc.
- **Mary Douglas,** Guest of Dr. Douglas
- **Mary Wright,** Program Director/Facilitator, The Conference Board
- **Melissa Dannenberg**
- **Melissa Reishus,** The Sea Glass Group
- **Michael Kinne,** President, IlliniCare
- **Michele Bromberg,** IL Nursing Practice Act Coordinator, IL Department of Financial & Professional Regulation, Division of Professional Regulation
- **Michelle Atkinson**
- **Mimi Alschuler,** Development Director, Access Living (VIP Reception Only)
- **Myra Glassman,** Member, Executive Board, SEIU Illinois Council, SEIU
- **Neil Anderson,** Physical Production, Operations, Access Living
- **Pam Capraro,** Manager, Vocational Rehab Center, Rehab Institute of Chicago
- **Parul Arora,** Senior Student Nurse, University of Illinois, College of Nursing
- **Patrick Maher,** Managing Director, nAblement; President, NSCIA
- **Patricia Sheahan,** Associate General Counsel, Rehabilitation Institute of Chicago
- **Patricia A. Shiu,** Director, DOL/Office of Federal Contract Compliance Programs (OFCCP)
- **Paul Siegel,** SEIU, Local 73, Division for Social Services
- **Peter Witzler,** SEIU
- **Rahnee Patrick,** Director of Independent Living, Access Living
- **Raymond Curry,** Dean for Education, Feinberg School of Medicine, Northwestern University
- **Rebecca Skipper,** Concepts, Inc.
- **Rene Luna,** Access Living
- **Richard L. Horne, EdD,** Division Director for Policy Planning and Research, DOL/ODEP
- **Robert Mendonsa,** CEO, Aetna Better Health, Illinois
- **Robin Jones,** Director & Instructor, DBTAC: Great Lakes ADA Center
- **Rodger DeRose,** CEO, Kessler Foundation
- **Rose Marie Toscano,** Co-Chair, Task Force; Professor, National Technical Institute for the Deaf/Rochester Institute of Technology, Task Force on Healthcare Careers for People who are DHH
- **Rosemary Ciotti, RN, MSN,** Board Member; Clinical Specialist/Nurse Practitioner, National Organization of Nurses with Disabilities
- **Sandy Hanebrink,** Occupational Therapist, Co-Author of "A Guide to Reasonable Accommodations for OT Practitioners with Disabilities"
- **Sarah Ailey,** Treasurer, National Organization of Nurses with Disabilities
- **Sheila Perkins,** VP, Employment Services, Chicago Lighthouse for People who are Blind and Visually Impaired
- **Sheila Romano,** Executive Director, ICDD; IL Council of Developmental Disabilities IL State Officials

- **Stanley Yarnell, MD,** Physician
- **Steve Pemberton,** Divisional VP of Diversity and Inclusion, Walgreen Co.
- **Sue Swenson,** Acting Director, National Institute on Disability and Rehabilitation Research (NIDRR), U.S. Department of Education
- **Susan Douglas, MD,** Public Policy Consultant
- **Susan O'Keefe,** Program Manager, Health Care Workforce Institute
- **Susanne Marie Bruyere,** National Employer Technical Assistance Center, Cornell University
- **Tamar Heller, PhD,** Professor/Head Department of Disability and Human Development/Director of the Institute on Disability and Human Development, University of Illinois at Chicago
- **Tari Hartman Squire,** Partner, EIN SOF
- **Terri Harkin,** SEIU
- **Vanessa Rivera,** VIP Reception Registration Volunteer, Access Living
- **Victor Rowley,** Stanley Yarnell's Aide
- **Yvette Crespo,** Director, RS Operations, Kaiser Permanente; Program Director, Project Search
- **Yvonne Tisdel,** Corporate VP, Human Resources & System Diversity, SSM Health Care
- **Zeferino Murillo,** Employment Coordinator, VR&E VetSuccess

Appendix B: Agenda

Health Care: Career Trends, Best Practices & Call-to-Action Summit
Tuesday, May 17, 2011
Access Living of Metropolitan Chicago

Agenda

8:00 – 9:00 AM	**Registration and Continental Breakfast**

9:00 – 9:30 AM	**Welcome (in order of appearance)**

- **Eric Grossman**, Access Living Chairman of the Board
- **Dr. Larry J. Goodman**, CEO Rush University Medical Center
- **Commissioner Karen Tamley**, City of Chicago Mayor's Office for People with Disabilities
- **Assistant Secretary Kathleen Martinez**, U.S. Department of Labor Office of Disability Employment Policy
- **Secretary Hilda L. Solis**, U.S. Department of Labor
- **Kareem Dale**, Special Assistant to the President for Disability Policy, The White House

9:30 – 10:30 AM	**Trends and Perspectives**

- **Martha Artiles**, Chief Diversity Officer, ManpowerGroup presents Manpower-National Council on Disability Report: Workforce Infrastructure in Support of People with Disabilities: Matching Human Resources to Service Needs.
- **Dr. Stanley Yarnell**, Retired Medical Director, Dept. of Rehabilitation, St. Mary's Medical Center, San Francisco and Clinical Associate Professor Emeritus, Dept. of Rehabilitation and Physical Medicine, Stanford University Medical School, 2011 recipient of St. Mary's "Pillar of St. Mary's Award" in California and former board member of the World Institute on Disability.

10:30 – 10:45 AM	**Break**

10:45 AM – 12:30 PM

- **Beth Marks**, RN, PhD, President, National Organization of Nurses with Disabilities. As a Research Associate Professor in the Department of Disability and Human Development, University of Illinois at Chicago and Associate Director for Research in the Rehabilitation Research and Training Center on Aging with Developmental Disabilities, she directs research programs on empowerment and advancement of persons with disabilities. She has published numerous articles and books related to health promotion and advocacy, and primary health care for people with disabilities. She will introduce the video "Open the Door, Get 'Em a Locker: Educating Nursing Students with Disabilities," that she co-produced with Dr. Bronwynne Evans.

Panel I: The Clinical Setting: New Strategies

- **Moderator: Dr. Kristi Kirschner**, MD, Professor at Northwestern University Feinberg School of Medicine in Clinical Medical Humanities and Bioethics and in Physical Medicine and Rehabilitation. She is an attending physician at Schwab Rehabilitation Hospital.
- **Panelists:**
  - **Bronwynne Evans**, PhD, RN, is an Associate Professor, a Fellow of both the American Academy of Nursing and the Academy of Nursing Education, and NIH-funded researcher in the College of Nursing & Health Innovation at Arizona State University. Nationally known for her work with American Indian and Hispanic/Latino students and students with disabilities, Dr. Evans has almost three decades of experience in nursing education, from associate degree to doctoral programs.
  - **Sandy Hanebrink**, OTR/L is the Branch Director of Touch the Future, Inc. in Anderson, SC. She is Chair of the Network of OT Practitioners with Disabilities and member of the AOTA Multi-culture Diversity and Inclusion Network.
  - **Rosemary Ciotti**, RN, MSN, CRNP, President of Accessible Living Inc., located in Arlington, Virginia where she primarily works with persons with spinal cord injuries in Community Health Nursing as a small business owner.
  - **Dr. Susan Douglas**, MD, JD, is from California and received her Juris Doctor Degree in 2007. She is a policy consultant and has worked as an independent advisor for the Affordable Care Act.

  Q & A with guest speakers from the audience

12:30 – 1: 30 PM	**Lunch** (Sponsored by National Organization of Nurses with Disabilities)
	Luncheon Speaker: Patricia A. Shiu, Director, U.S. Department of Labor (DOL) Office of Federal Contract Compliance Programs (OFCCP)
1:30 – 2:45 PM	**Panel II: Career Opportunities: Growth in Demand**

- **Moderator: Dr. Brigida Hernandez**, PhD, Director of Research, YAI Network, New York, NY. Research Assistant Professor in the Department of Disability and Human Development at the University of Illinois at Chicago.

- **Panelists:**
  - **Yvette Crespo**, from California, is certified in HR Management, and is Kaiser Permanente's Director of National Recruitment Systems and Operations and Project SEARCH Program Director.
  - **David Mulvey**, MSW, Service Coordinator Tri-Counties Regional Center, Board Member Service Employees International Union (SEIU) Local 721, Chair SEIU California Committee on Developmental Disabilities.
  - **Kevin Shanklin**, MBA, Executive Director in the Office of the President and CEO of Blue Cross Blue Shield Association in Chicago, Illinois.

  Q & A with guest speakers from the audience

- **Karen McCulloh**, RN, BS, Healthcare Summit Subject Matter Expert; Co-Founder, and Immediate Past President of the National Organization of Nurses with Disabilities.

2:45 – 3:00 PM   **Summary & Closing Remarks**

- **Assistant Secretary Kathleen Martinez**, U. S. Department of Labor Office of Disability Employment Policy
  - Video, "I Can," a public service announcement produced by the U.S. Department of Labor Office of Disability Employment Policy

3:00 PM   **Adjourn**

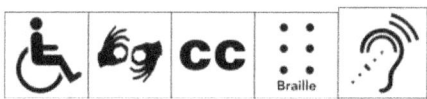

Access Living of Metropolitan Chicago wishes to thank the National Organization of Nurses with Disabilities, The Chicago Lighthouse for People Who are Blind or Visually Impaired and the Westin Chicago River North Hotel

Appendix C: Workforce Infrastructure in Support of People with Disabilities: Matching Human Resources to Service Needs

Executive Summary

Americans with disabilities depend on the disability services infrastructure, which consists of health, education, and social services programs. The need for these services is expected to increase significantly in the coming decades as a result of several factors, most notably the aging of the baby boom generation and declining birthrates. These trends threaten the future availability and quality of services for people with disabilities. As the threat grows, so do the downsides to the American economy and society, which are increasingly engaged competitively on a global basis. People with disabilities occupy a strategic place in America's ability to compete. Either their talents and ambitions will be developed into a resource for our society, or they will remain on the margins, battling for shrinking resources. This report from the National Council on Disability (NCD) presents recommendations (with a rationale for each) that call for partnerships among federal departments and agencies, their State counterparts, and the private sector, including organizations involved with education/training, health care, and employment services. A concerted effort is needed by these sectors to ensure that the projected shortfall in the workforce of the disability services infrastructure entities can be quickly overcome. Unless everyone works together to meet this goal, the quality of life for people with disabilities will be threatened. The gains made over the past two decades in the levels at which people with disabilities participate socially and economically will be lost, and achieving levels of independence comparable to those of people who are not disabled will be pushed farther into the future. The national health care debate, so much a part of the political scene in 2009, as well as the stimulus funds made available by the Obama Administration and Congress, create a unique opportunity to focus attention on the current and future needs of people with disabilities. The potential for refocusing priorities to ensure that the resources are available in the critical areas of employment, education, and health care services for people with disabilities is great and must be realized.

Numerous forecasts based on diverse trends all point to a shortage of qualified workers to meet the needs of people who are disabled. NCD calls for policymakers at all levels of government to proactively address these shortages and examine how labor market changes are driving both current and future supply needs. This six-section report covers the following topics:

1. Introduction and background
2. National trends, gaps and barriers, and their implications for people with disabilities and the disability services industry
3. Disability services infrastructure occupations: supply and demand
4. Private sector strategies for building and maintaining a sufficient supply of disability infrastructure occupations
5. Public sector strategies for building and maintaining a sufficient supply of disability infrastructure occupations

6.   Recommendations

Section 1 outlines the strategies used to examine the current and future supply and demand associated with labor markets of the disability services infrastructure. This examination began by identifying organizations and government agencies serving people with disabilities to determine what services currently exist. An extensive literature search identified the best available sources regarding disability service worker shortages and gaps in service delivery. Information from the Bureau of Labor Statistics (BLS) of the U.S. Department of Labor was used to identify specific occupations and future projections. While existing resources help identify trends affecting the demand for future disability services and workers, the supply side has a dearth of resources, requiring more extrapolation and development. The model described in this section and detailed throughout the report provides an expanded research foundation that can be further developed through successive iterations into a tool for guiding policy formation.

Section 2 reviews issues and trends relative to skill shortages in the disability-related service industry as examined by Manpower Inc., including the aging baby boom generation and declining U.S. birthrates. The baby boomers are beginning to retire, thus increasing demands on health care, mobility support, and other services. These demands will generate further restrictions on services available to people with disabilities. This section lays the foundation for the first iteration of a more robust approach to project demand for disability services, which is a key unmet need in policy formation.

Section 3 summarizes data currently available from the Employment Outlook Projections of the BLS related to the supply-demand gap in disability-related occupations. According to the BLS, many infrastructure occupations are projected to be in high demand, particularly those associated with health care. This section suggests ways to increase the supply of disability services infrastructure workers using promising recruiting and retention practices such as increasing salaries and benefits, training to upgrade worker skills, recruiting workers from underutilized populations, and leveraging transferable skills. By developing the discussion of the supply-demand gap and exploring best practices to reduce the gap, this section lays the foundation for a supply management discipline. Such a discipline is mandatory to formulate disability services policy, especially on the national level, where supply management has been conspicuous in its absence.

Section 4 explores recruiting and retention strategies used in the private sector. Public policy affecting the disability services infrastructure cannot be developed in isolation from the private sector. When employers explore current and future workforce demographics to develop workforce management strategies, they are engaging in the private sector version of disability services supply management. Using their data and tools, employers can better identify and target appropriate candidates for disability service positions. These private sector practices provide models and strategies that the public sector can apply as well. In fact, as employers implement workforce management, they may interface with parallel public sector programs. Employers can work with community-based rehabilitation programs and vocational rehabilitation agencies to develop and tap underutilized populations. Such partnerships offer employers a large pool of potential job candidates that can receive job training through vocational services. Another useful strategy employers can explore relates to the successful return to work of injured/ill workers and the prevention of disabilities. Some employers, for example, may develop or hire return-to-work coordinators and case managers to facilitate return to work. Such private sector efforts offer a laboratory for disability services strategies and can provide some of the needed infrastructure that must be addressed through public policy.

Section 5 explores ways in which the public sector can work with the private sector to provide a suitable workforce infrastructure for people with disabilities. Public agencies and programs can establish practices that promote an adequate supply of qualified frontline workers. These public agencies and programs include the State-federal vocational rehabilitation services system, the Department of Veterans Affairs, the Workforce Investment Act and One-Stop Centers, and the Ticket to Work Program. This section also examines how new technologies and Web-enabled tools can improve access to services and information for people with disabilities. In another important discussion, this section identifies problems in health care supply and access for people with disabilities. Proposed solutions in health care reform include the medical home model, with primary care physicians coordinating all care, and electronic medical records to improve efficiency of delivery. In another strategic discussion, the section explores the need for transition services for youth with disabilities that could be met through the postsecondary education system. U.S. community colleges can provide an efficient and accessible link between students and their careers through career and technical education.

Section 6 highlights the recommendations that flow from the discussions in the previous sections. These recommendations include how private sector employers can improve their hiring and retention practices to ensure an adequate supply of workers; how federal and State agencies can target service strategies to enhance the supply of workers; how we can redirect resources in our educational and training establishments to focus on infrastructure occupations; and what we can do to monitor workforce supply and demand so that planning can accommodate unexpected events and redirect resources accordingly.

The appendices provide detailed evidence that supports the findings in each of the sections and the recommendations. An extensive search of the literature was conducted, and many of the documents that provided an empirical basis for this report have been abstracted and placed in Appendix A. Readers who wish to have more detailed information can review these abstracts, which are grouped according to report section. Appendix B contains detailed information and charts on many disability services infrastructure occupations. This information provided the basis for section 3; it is also useful for program planning and as guidance for schools and training programs that offer career and vocational counseling for their students.

All these discussions identify opportunities for public-private sector partnerships to help implement public policy to better manage the nation's disability services infrastructure. Given the overlap between private and public goals and programs, such partnerships are inevitable. This public-private overlap is significant for policy formulation and implementation, because it is based on an even more significant underlying connection. People with disabilities have a shared interest with their nation and government in resolving challenges to disability services infrastructure management; in fact, this population contains an untapped resource to realize a solution to this policy challenge.

Appendix D: Exploring the Bottom Line: The Costs and Benefits of Workers with Disabilities in the Health Care Sector

Summary

Employment struggles experienced by the disability community are well-documented. Although employers seem receptive to hiring individuals with disabilities, they are concerned with the bottom line: Will the benefits associated with this workforce outweigh the costs? To date, research of employers who have hired adults with various types of disabilities has found favorable views. However, such employer data have been primarily anecdotal and subjective in nature. In a groundbreaking study, DePaul University researchers examined the costs and benefits of workers with disabilities using both subjective (qualitative) and objective (quantitative) data.

Study 1: A focus group was held with 12 administrators from 7 large hospitals representing the Chicagoland area to discuss their experiences with the disabled workforce. Focus group findings revealed the following themes:

(1) <u>Disability employment agencies</u> and <u>champions</u> were critical for recruiting, hiring, & building corporate culture.
(2) <u>Frontline managers</u> were viewed as having biases and concerns with job performance and costs.
(3) <u>Promotion opportunities</u> were limited, with many holding semi-skilled positions (clerical, food service, laundry).
(4) <u>Costs</u> were viewed as minimal and worth the expense.
(5) <u>Benefits</u> included dedicated and reliable employees and a diverse workforce.

Study 2: Eight Chicagoland hospitals participated in a study that compared the work-related variables (i.e., tenure, absenteeism, job performance, supervision, worker's compensation claims, and accommodations) of workers with (n=45) and without (n=81) disabilities holding comparable positions. We learned that healthcare workers with disabilities <u>held a variety of positions</u>: 33% Administrative Support Workers, 29% Professionals, 11% Officials and Managers, 11% Technicians, 11% Service Workers, and 4% Other. A review of HR records indicated that workers with and without disabilities had <u>similar</u> (1) <u>job performance</u> and (2) <u>amount of supervision required</u> ratings. The number of documented <u>accommodations</u> requests and <u>costs</u> were minimal: 15 requests, <u>averaged $521</u>. Areas where workers with disabilities <u>did not fare as well</u> included <u>tenure</u>, <u>unscheduled absences</u>, and to a lesser extent number of <u>worker's compensation claims</u>.

Although findings from Study 2 are noteworthy, generalizations should be made with caution given that this is a first attempt to directly compare HR data of both workforces (disabled and non-disabled) and participating hospitals represented the Chicago region. With those caveats in mind, the following implications are presented:
(1) Need for more accurate data on workers with disabilities (e.g., overall representation, types of positions held).

(2) Need to expand recruitment efforts beyond disability employment agencies (e.g., professional communities).
(3) Need to educate employers with quantitative data that are comparable to the non-disabled workforce.
(4) Need to reach out to frontline management to combat potential biases.
(5) Need to foster professional growth and promotion opportunities.
(6) Need to reinforce low cost of accommodations and benefits to entire workforce (e.g., flexible work schedules).

This three-year project (2004-2007) was conducted in collaboration with:
- DePaul University
- *disabilityworks*
- IL Department of Commerce and Economic Opportunity
- Mayor's Office of Workforce Development
- Chicagoland Chamber of Commerce
- Mayor's Office for People with Disabilities

References: Hernandez, B., & McDonald, K. (2010). The costs and benefits of workers with disabilities. *Journal of Rehabilitation, 76*, 15-23.
Hernandez, B., McDonald, K., Divilbiss, M., Horin, E., Velcoff, J., & Donoso, O. (2008). Reflections on the disabled workforce: Focus groups with healthcare, hospitality, and retail administrators. *Employee Responsibilities and Rights Journal, 20*, 157-164.

Contact: Brigida Hernandez, PhD
Director of Research
YAI Network (New York, New York)
brigida.hernandez@yai.org